Unplug

Unplug

How to Survive and Thrive
In a Wi-Fi World Gone Wild

Sam Wieder

Unplug
How to Survive and Thrive in a Wi-Fi World Gone Wild
By Sam Wieder

New Energy Dynamics
Post Office Box 963
Greensburg, PA 15601

This material is not intended to replace medical advice but to supplement regular care by your physician. Every effort has been made to ensure the accuracy of the information in this book as of the date of publication. The author assumes no responsibility for how readers use this information, or for any circumstances arising out of the use, misuse, interpretation or application of any information supplied.

Library of Congress Cataloging-in-Publication Data

Wieder, Sam
Unplug: how to survive and thrive in a wi-fi world gone wild/by Sam Wieder—1st ed.
ISBN: 978-1-892241-03-0

To Jacqueline,
who opened me to a world of possibility

Contents

Acknowledgements

I gratefully acknowledge those who have aided me on the journey of discovery that led to the writing of this book, as well as those who offered their feedback and support through the writing process.

To Ann Louise Gittleman, whose book Zapped awakened me to the dangers of electromagnetic radiation and motivated me to start taking them seriously.

To Sal La Duca, the environmental consultant and building biologist who educated me about my household electrical issues and guided me through the process of creating a more environmentally friendly home and office. Sal's depth of knowledge about electrical science is truly astounding, only exceeded by his generosity in sharing his expertise and his passion for helping people live more safely in our electromagnetic world.

To William Strunk, Jr. and E.B. White, whose time-honored classic The Elements of Style not only offered me sound advice on how to write clear, potent sentences but showed me how a small book could make a big difference.

To my colleagues and fellow professional speakers in the National Speakers Association, who have shown me the power of using personal stories to educate, illuminate, and motivate just about anyone.

To Doug Hagy, the first reader of this book, whose familiarity and experience with my topic enabled him to provide me with some invaluable initial feedback.

To my niece Megan Wieder, a talented writer who read my manuscript when I thought it was complete and opened my mind to a major possibility for improvement that I wouldn't have seen otherwise.

Introduction

Are you feeling stressed, tired, or run down far too often? If so, do you ever wonder why?

We are now living in an age in which rapidly advancing technology has, in so many ways, made life easier than it has ever been. Our kitchens are equipped with a variety of time-saving appliances. Our offices contain the latest productivity-boosting computer equipment. We can harness the power of the Internet to quickly and easily communicate with one another and access a world of information. Through wireless technology, we can also take this communication power with us wherever we go, whether we are making a call from a cell phone or possibly using that phone, a laptop computer, or electronic tablet to connect with the Internet through a wi-fi network.

With all of this convenience, speed, and power at our command, you might think that this would allow us to embrace a more relaxed approach to life than that of previous generations. In fact, though, our love affair with technology seems to be having just the opposite effect.

While we can instantly send email messages to hundreds of people at a time, we also face the burden of processing or responding to the multitude of messages that we receive. While the Internet gives us access to a treasure trove of information, this wonderland of knowledge can also be an entrancing distraction from the priorities in our lives. While cell phones give us the ability to stay in touch with friends, family, and business contacts wherever we go, they also give others the ability to reach us 24 hours a day, even at times when we'd rather not be reached.

Technology was designed to serve us—and it certainly does in so many ways. But as it has become a bigger and bigger part of our lives, it often seems as if we have become a slave to this servant.

We have come to rely on technology to function in today's world. Yet, if we are not careful, that reliance can go beyond harnessing the power of a useful tool. It can assume the form of an addiction, one that continually lures us to our computers, cell phones, and other electronic gadgets, just so we can stay connected to the world and keep pace with the accelerating speed of life.

Of course, this need to keep pace and compulsion to interact with our technology creates a certain amount of psychological stress, which in turn can have a negative impact on our health. What relatively few people stop to consider, however, is how spending so much time with our electronic gadgetry may also threaten our health on a more basic physical level.

Our electrical and electronic devices all generate an invisible electromagnetic field. Our bodies are also highly electrical and readily conduct radiation at a wide range of frequencies. Thus, when you spend more and more time with your electronic devices, engulfed in the radiation that they generate, you are conducting an electrical experiment and you are the subject.

If, indeed, electromagnetic radiation is a stressor to your body, we are now living in an age in which the magnitude of this stress is expanding at an accelerating pace. Since personal computers were first sold to a mass market in the last part of the 20th century, we have been swept up in an ongoing technology boom. As soon as one wave of technology is embraced by the public, another seems to emerge to replace it.

Our ever-expanding use of computers and digital electronics also places added demands on our electrical grid, demands that it wasn't designed to meet. As a result, the wiring in our homes, schools, and offices has become a greater source of radiation than ever before.

Add to all of this the rapid spread of radio frequency radiation. Since cell phones first came onto the market in the 1980's, they went from being a novel product idea to a communication tool used by millions of people worldwide. The U.S. alone now has nearly a quarter million cell phone antennas beaming their microwave radiation to the vast number of cell phones in use. When switched on, the cell phones themselves also radiate waves from all sides in order to receive signals from and send signals to a base station or antenna.

Electrical utility companies are also taking advantage of wireless technology by replacing traditional analog meters with digital "smart meters" that can transmit information about electrical usage, eliminating the need to send out meter readers to gather it. In addition, a growing number of homes, offices, restaurants, and hotels are making use of microwave-generating wi-fi networks to allow for wireless Internet access.

Electromagnetic radiation is now filling our world. Being invisible and undetectable to most people, it may seem harmless enough. But is it? Or might the rapid transformation of our natural world into one that is teaming with unnatural, man-made radiation be steadily and silently assaulting our health in ways that will only become widely recognized as time unfolds?

To shed some light on this question, I'd like to share my story.

Our technological powers increase, but the side effects
and potential hazards also escalate.

Alvin Toffler
Author of *Future Shock*

Chapter One

Venturing into the High-Tech Jungle

Early in my career, in August 1984, I landed a job as a marketing analyst. My job involved sitting at a typewriter all day, writing analytical marketing reports.

Naturally, I took great care in typing each sentence. I knew, after all, that if I hit the wrong key or mistyped a word, I would have to stop and use the correction ribbon to correct my mistake. And if, for some reason, the flow of my writing went astray or I made too many mistakes, I'd have to pull out the page, insert a clean sheet of paper, and start all over again. Like many writers before me, though, I simply accepted all of this as part of the writing process.

Then one day, there was some buzz around the office. The company was looking into investing in the latest emerging technology, a networked computer system. Soon I said goodbye to my typewriter and was working at my own personal computer. Suddenly, the process of writing had changed forever.

No longer did I have to type so gingerly in fear of making a mistake that I'd have to stop to correct. I could type away with speed and confidence, knowing that I could correct any mistakes with ease. Now, I also had a whole new degree of power over my writing. I could easily insert or replace words wherever needed. I could move sentences or whole paragraphs. I could save and file useful material I had written for one report so that it could be simply dropped into a similar type of report in the future.

With all of this new power, I wondered how I had ever been able to write anything worthwhile without a computer. I felt like a kid who had been given an exciting new toy, marveling at all I could do with it. As time passed, however, my excitement began to fade along with my energy. I continued to appreciate how much easier my computer had made my work, as well as how much it had expanded my creative flexibility. Still, there was just something about staring at a computer screen for 8 or more hours a day that seemed to sap my energy and cloud my thinking.

After awhile, I felt like I was running an ultra-marathon, the miles taking their toll, my energy steadily fading. At times, when a flood of new urgent assignments would land upon my desk, I'd somehow find a way to pick up the pace. Spending even more time at my computer, I'd attack my work with heightened intensity, pushing my endurance to the limit. While I was often amazed at how much I was able to accomplish during these bursts of effort, this only further depleted my energy reserves. Soon, I was once again dragging, doing the survivor's shuffle in a race that had no finish line.

Fortunately, after a few years, someone came to my rescue. I started dating a chiropractor named Jacqueline. Aside from adding some excitement to my personal life and introducing me to the rejuvenating power of chiropractic, Jacqueline helped me to see how different elements in my working environment might be wearing me down from one day to the next. For so long, I hadn't given any thought to how my office environment might be affecting the way that I felt. But if there were some simple changes I could make in my office that would help bring me back to life, I was only too eager to make them.

Following Jacqueline's advice, I then took steps to reshape and de-stress my office. I adjusted my office chair to provide proper support for my spine and lessen the stress on my body. I propped up my computer monitor on a few phone books so that I no longer had to hunch forward to look at my screen. I brought in a lamp with an incandescent daylight bulb to use as my main source of office lighting and kept the overhead fluorescent lights turned off.

Of all the changes I made in my office, altering my lighting seemed to have the most immediate impact. Switching to softer, incandescent lighting and eliminating those unforgiving fluorescent beams from above, I could instantly feel the difference. It was as if my whole office had been transformed from a police interrogation room into a peaceful and nurturing creative studio.

Finally, I was the master of my working environment—or so it seemed. While I felt somewhat better after addressing different issues that had been sapping my energy, I was still sitting behind a desk staring at a computer screen for hour after hour each day. As I ploughed through my work, my energy slid into a black hole while my mind felt like it was being engulfed by a pea soup fog. The only way to recover from this sorry state, it seemed, was to get away from my computer.

While this job served to pay my bills and helped to hone my writing skills, the excitement in my life came from what I did outside of the office. My dream was to one day work in the field of personal development as an inspirational speaker, writer, and success coach. So when I wasn't writing marketing reports, I was steadily taking steps to prepare myself for this career move.

I developed my public speaking skills by advancing through the Toastmasters International educational program. I completed advanced coaching and training skills certification programs. I also had a part-time job for a couple of years as a high school speech and debate coach.

Finally, I left my writing job and launched my own professional speaking and coaching business. When I made this move, I felt reborn. No longer was I staring at a computer screen all day, pushing myself to crank out one report after another. Instead, I was out speaking to groups, interacting with people, and rediscovering the excitement of connecting with the world of the living.

Naturally, this new business life had its own stresses. Still, the energy drain and mental fogginess that I had experienced by spending so much time at a computer seemed to just magically melt away. This gave me hope that I could leave all of that behind me forever.

***

Now my life was moving in a new and exciting direction. In addition to making a major career move, I also married Jacqueline, the wonderful woman who had helped to bring me back to life during the final years at my writing job. Since her work as a healer was all about helping people to rediscover their natural health and vitality, I couldn't have asked for a better life partner.

After we had been married for 10 years, we moved out of our apartment and into a spacious house, which we transformed into both a living and working environment. At one end of the house was a bright room with a big picture window, which looked out upon a backyard landscaped with reddish brown Japanese maple trees, beds of Black-eyed Susans, two plump, green fir trees, two sprawling red maple trees, and a backdrop of a few towering Norway Spruce. The room overlooking this cascade of nature became the office and treatment room for Jacqueline's chiropractic and natural healing practice. Accented by its picturesque view and brightened with natural sunlight, this room offered the perfect setting for healing work.

At the opposite end of the house was a spacious room that became my coaching and consulting room. This room had two windows, a large picture window on the sunny front side of the house and a smaller 3-panel window on the shady side of the house. With an adjustable vertical window blind on both the front and side windows, I could easily adjust the amount and intensity of energizing sunlight streaming into the room.

Across the hall from my coaching room was a cozy, somewhat smaller room that became our joint home office. This room had a picture window that looked out upon rhododendron plants up close to the house and a giant white pine tree and spreading magnolia tree several feet out. We also invited wildlife into this view by setting up a bird feeder pole with two hanging feeders. This not only attracted a variety of local birds but occasionally provided us with a source of entertainment when squirrels would leap from the nearby rhododendrons to latch onto the feeders as well.

To make this office the command center for our two businesses, we packed in our computers and office equipment and furniture in a way that flowed and allowed for easy access to almost anything we needed. Overall, the room had the look and feel of the bridge on the Starship Enterprise, even though we weren't soaring through space.

Our overall goal for the house was to make it a healthy and supportive environment in which to live and work. We did this by supplementing the natural light with daylight and/or full-spectrum light bulbs and fixtures. We installed a reverse-osmosis water filtering system to provide us with clean drinking water and added a filter to the showerhead to filter out chlorine. We had an environmental testing firm evaluate the air quality in the house and used room air filters to help purify the air. We even brought in a feng shui consultant to show us what we could do to optimize the energy flow and harmony within our home.

After doing all of this, we felt that we were finally set. We had plenty of space in which to live and run our home-based businesses. There was also an expansiveness about the house that felt liberating after coming from many years of apartment living. As a result, we both felt more open to attracting new possibilities into our lives, ready to explore how we might make a bigger impact in the world, all while being grounded in a home base that we had made our own.

Our highest intentions for our new home were best summarized by the following framed verse, which we hung near the front door.

> May this home be
> a place of happiness
> and health,
> of contentment,
> generosity and hope,
> a home of creativity
> and kindness.
> May those who visit
> and those who live here
> know only blessing and peace.

Soon we were swept up in the flow of our professional lives. When Jacqueline wasn't treating patients, she was teaching healthcare seminars around the country. In addition to helping her coordinate those seminars, I also stepped up my own business activities, teaching business communication classes at the local college, chairing a big one-day educational event for my National Speakers Association chapter, leading business mastermind groups, and serving as president of my networking group. It seemed that we had become the quintessential professional power couple—a dynamic duo that couldn't be stopped.

I must admit, though, that there were times during that first year in our new home that I felt like I was running on fumes. I was excited about the things that I was doing and drew upon that excitement to drive myself forward. It just felt like underneath that mantle of excitement I was a man who was barely holding himself together.

These feelings of fragility became more and more frequent as the year wore on. Then, as the year drew to a close, my overall energy plummeted. I was spent.

Finally recognizing that I wasn't unstoppable, I cut back on my activities and commitments as I entered the new year. My body was clearly telling me that if I didn't slow down, I would totally fall apart. And since it felt like I was right on the edge of this actually happening, this was a message that I couldn't ignore.

For awhile, I only did what was absolutely necessary to run my business. Soon, though, even that was too much for me. I went through the motions of working, but I had little or nothing to show for my efforts. My working life was like a slow-motion movie that I simply couldn't speed up. Dragging me down was a persistent exhausted feeling, accompanied by an unrelenting pressure in my chest.

I had felt traces of this chest pressure from time to time during the previous year when I was taking on the world, most notably when I was working at my computer. Somehow, though, I had always seemed able to push through that feeling to accomplish whatever task I was tackling. But this time, that just didn't seem possible.

Out of necessity, I finally decided to take a break from my business and focus on regaining my health. Instead of sitting at my computer in my home office for so much of the day, I escaped this environment of technology by spending more and more time in other rooms that were more peaceful and nurturing. I also made a point of regularly going outside for fresh air and sunshine.

I felt fortunate that my wife Jacqueline was a holistic healer, since she gave me treatments to help me regain my health. But I also needed to play an important role in my own recovery, which I did through resting, meditating, and eating a healthy diet. After several months of healthcare and extreme self-care, the ongoing pressure in my chest finally dissolved, my energy returned, and it seemed that once more I would be able to resume a normal, healthy, productive life.

As I moved on with my life, however, it wasn't quite the free and easy ride I had hoped it would be. Every so often, seemingly out of nowhere, I would be stricken with all of the debilitating symptoms I had suffered through during my year-long bout with chronic fatigue. The pressure in my chest returned. I felt exhausted and unable to focus. The whole world seemed overwhelming. At times, it even felt like I wanted to jump out of my skin.

When all of these symptoms hit, I would turn again to my holistic healer wife for help. She would then work her healing magic on me and before long I'd be feeling better.

It was only a matter of time, though, before my symptoms would return and I'd have to once again turn to my wife to come to my rescue.

This alternating pattern between feeling good and feeling stressed out or exhausted continued for several years, giving me the sense that this was just the way my life was going to be.

As time passed, my wife Jacqueline's health and well-being was also on an ongoing rollercoaster ride. She would feel fine for a while. Then, out of nowhere, one health issue or another would pop up to slow her down or keep her in bed for a day or two.

Often her physical ailments were accompanied by bouts of depression. To escape the blues, she would distract herself by sitting at her computer in the evening and working through the online version of the New York Times crossword puzzle. She might also do some online research for her wellness newsletter or write emails to her network of friends and professional colleagues across the country.

These distractions helped Jacqueline to shift her attention away from how bad she was feeling. Still, she always eventually had to face up to her health challenges and find her way back to wellness.

Somehow we had gone from being an unstoppable power couple to a husband and wife team whose health cycled up and down like a never-ending rollercoaster. Why was this happening? We ate a healthy diet. We got regular chiropractic adjustments to keep our bodies in balance. We had taken steps to make our home a haven for health. Yet, for some reason, we never seemed to be able to stay healthy and were always left wondering when our health and energy would once again start to slip away.

This is what our life was like for many years. Then, entering the year 2010, Jacqueline's health challenges started to accelerate. That whole year for her was a downward slide. Too sick to continue seeing patients by mid-fall, she finally closed her chiropractic practice. From that point on, her condition only got worse and worse. After then enduring 6 weeks of ongoing pain and suffering, including a stressful stint in the hospital, her body could take no more. On December 13th, she passed away.

I was numb. The love of my life was gone. After 20 years of marriage, it was hard to imagine my life without Jacqueline in it. But now, suddenly, that was exactly the life that lay ahead of me, a life without my partner, my help mate, my health mate, my soul mate.

***

A month later, I was in our home office one day when a book on Jacqueline's desk caught my eye. Its bright orange dust jacket was so striking that I was surprised I hadn't noticed it before. After picking up the book and glancing at the cover, I was immediately captivated by its bold, one-word title—Zapped. Then, as I looked more closely at the cover, I could almost hear Jacqueline's voice whispering inside my head, "Read this book, Sam." So I did.

The author, Ann Louise Gittleman, described how she had been troubled with a wide variety of baffling and unrelenting health issues for many years. Then, she was diagnosed with a benign tumor of the parotid, a salivary gland located just below the earlobe. As this was a rare tumor, typically caused by radiation exposure, neither she nor her doctor could figure out what might have caused it.

After all, she didn't live or work near a nuclear power plant and rarely had medical x-rays or other screening tests.

This mystery, though, got Gittleman to consider another possibility. What if her health issues were caused by something she was exposed to every day, something she had considered harmless? As she then took a closer look at her life, the clues to solving this mystery fell into place.

A prolific writer, she spent a lot of her time either writing at her computer or traveling to promote her books, talking on a cell phone in cars, planes, and trains. It seemed that she had become a victim of these radiating tools of her trade. Researching this matter further, she uncovered mounting evidence of the health risks of prolonged exposure to radiation from common electrical appliances and electronic equipment, particularly seemingly harmless wireless devices such as cell phones and wireless (wi-fi) computer routers.

This, in turn, led her to write her book Zapped, which describes how to minimize the health threats posed by the electromagnetic pollution in our everyday lives.

As I pondered Gittleman's story, I began to wonder—could the health mystery that she had unraveled be the same one that had baffled us for so many years? It seemed that we had done almost everything to make our home a healthy place in which to live and work. Yet, the one thing that we hadn't fully considered, researched, understood, or addressed was the health impact of the technology that was a part of our everyday lives.

Suddenly, this whole subject fascinated me. Eager to learn more, I devoured the rest of Gittleman's book like I might a compelling mystery novel. As I read, it was as if a door had swung open to an unseen world I had never thought to explore.

In the past, I had never had any great interest in science. Now, though, that began to change, as I discovered how a deeper understanding of biology and electromagnetism might very well hold the key to reclaiming my health and living a long, productive life. This, in turn, set me on the path to learn all that I could about the biological effects of man-made radiation.

Let me share with you the essence of what I learned.

Chapter Two

Illuminating the Unknown

Long before man learned how to generate and harness the power of electricity to light up and electrify the world, there was an abundance of electricity already at work. This was the natural flow of electrical impulses within the human body. Through the communication network of the nervous system, the brain is constantly sending and receiving these impulses to orchestrate the body's many functions. These electrical signals, in fact, are what enable us to walk and talk, to keep our hearts beating, and to mobilize the chemicals needed to help us heal when we are hurt or respond to the dangers in our environment.

The human body is also an efficient conductor of electricity and can act as an effective antenna to attract energy from its surroundings. Whenever you are exposed to an electromagnetic field, whether you are opening your refrigerator door or typing away at your computer keyboard, your body absorbs that field like a paper towel soaks up water. The question is: what, if any, effect does this have on the body?

Many Ways You're Harmed by Unseen Rays

The harmful effects of high-frequency ionizing radiation are widely recognized. Exposure to ultraviolet light, for instance, can lead to sunburn if the exposure is fairly brief. Even more exposure could result in the development of skin cancer or cataracts.

But what about exposure to radiation from such sources cell phones, computers, and electrical appliances? Since radiation from these sources is insufficient to heat human tissue, some scientists have concluded that it has little or no effect on the body. A mounting volume of evidence, however, is emerging to show otherwise. Here is a small sampling of that evidence and its implications:

DNA Damage: Twenty minutes of exposure to cell-phone radiation has been found to break double strands of DNA. If this damage continues at a rate faster than the body can repair, this could lead to the development of cancer.[1]

Assault to the Brain: Exposure to mobile phone radiation has been found to create leakage in the blood-brain barrier. This allows neurotoxins in the bloodstream to flow into the brain, which over time could lead to brain cell death and the formation of tumors, as well as Alzheimer's and early dementia.[2]

Inflammatory Diseases: Electromagnetic exposure leads to elevated levels of calcium within cells, which in turn results in the production of a compound called peroxynitrite. This compound is a major cause of most inflammatory diseases, including neurodegenerative and cardiovascular diseases, migraines, and allergies.[3]

---

[1] A. Campisi et al, "Reactive oxygen species levels and DNA fragmentation on astrocytes in primary culture after acute exposure to low intensity microwave electromagnetic field," *Neuroscience Letters,* vol. 473 (2010): 52-55.

[2] L.G. Salford et al, "Nerve cell damage in mammalian brain after exposure to microwaves from GSM mobile phones, *"Environmental Health Perspectives,"* vol. 111, no. 7, (2003).

[3] M. Pall, "Electromagnetic Fields act via activation of voltage-gated calcium channels to produce beneficial or adverse effects," *Journal of Cellular and Molecular Medicine,* 6-26-2013.

Learning Disabilities and Loss of Concentration:
Suzanne Bawin found that modulated radio frequency radiation can remove calcium ions from cell membranes in the brain, making the membranes more prone to leakage. This can spark the nerve cells to overstimulate the brain, making it difficult for a person to concentrate and setting the stage for Attention Deficit Hyperactive Disorder.[4]

Decreased Fertility: Researchers find that sperm quality and motility is diminished when men wear a cell phone, PDA, or pager on their belt or in their pants pocket.[5]

Melatonin Suppression and Weakened Immune System: By 2000, there were 15 studies showing that exposure to various common types of electromagnetic radiation suppresses the body's ability to produce melatonin. This vital hormone not only helps to regulate sleep patterns but is a powerful antioxidant that boosts your immune system and defends against cancer.[6]

Decrease in Insulin/Increase in Blood Sugar:
A 1994 study by Navakatikian revealed that radio frequency radiation created a significant drop in insulin in test subjects. Suppressed insulin, over time, can lead to high blood sugar, obesity, and diabetes.[7]

---

[4] S.M. Bawin et al, "Effects of modulated VHF fields on the central nervous system," *Academy of Science,* 247: 74-81.

[5] A. Agarwal et. al, "Effect of cell phone usage on semen analysis in men attending infertility clinic: an observational study," *Fertility and Sterility,* vol. 92, no. 1, (2008): 124-128.

[6] Neil Cherry, "EMR reduces Melatonin in Animals and People," July 26, 2000, http://www.feb.se/EMFguru/Research/emf-emr/EMR-Reduces-Melatonin.htm.

[7] Navakatikian, MA & Tomashevskaya, LA, 1994, "Phasic Behavioral and Endocrine Effects of Microwaves of Non-Thermal Intensity," *Biological Effects of Electric and Magnetic Fields,* Carpenter DO (Ed), Academic Press, pp. 333-342.

Mounting Evidence of a Growing Danger

As the world has become electrified and filled with a wide variety of radiation-producing appliances and devices, a number of epidemiological studies have been conducted to examine the possible effects of this on our population.

Among the most ground-breaking studies were those done by Dr. Samuel Milham, a pioneering physician-epidemiologist, specializing in studying the health effects of electricity. In comparing disease and mortality statistics before and after the electrification of the United States, Milham made an interesting observation. When rural or agricultural areas of the country became electrified, rates of cardiovascular and degenerative diseases began to rise, eventually matching the previously higher rates of urban areas, where electricity had been introduced much earlier.

In studying health and occupational data, Milham discovered a much higher than average incidence of cancer and other degenerative diseases among workers who were exposed to high levels of electromagnetic fields. These included power line men, firefighters, aluminum reduction plant workers, as well as typists and office workers.

Beyond examining data about population segments that had high exposure to electromagnetic fields, Milham also looked at a group that had avoided the movement toward electrification. He observed that the Old Order Amish, who prohibit all use of electricity, have very low rates of neurodegenerative disease and lower rates of heart disease and diabetes than the overall population.

Also seeing the Amish as an excellent case study group, Dr. Judith Westman studied the death rates from cancer in the Ohio Amish. Publishing her findings in 2009, Westman reported that the Ohio Amish had a remarkable

40% lower incidence of all cancers than other residents of the state. She also noted that the Old Order Amish population's avoidance of electricity was the only significant element of their lifestyle that could account for this result.[8]

Many researchers have uncovered a link between exposure to electromagnetic fields (EMFs) and disease. A 2007 review of 16 studies of the EMF/cancer link showed an increased risk of brain tumors among cell phone users. This data revealed that those using cell phones for 10 years and longer had a 240% increased risk, on average, of developing an ipsilateral glioma tumor on the same side of the head that the phone was used.[9]

A 2009 multinational study also found that people who used cell phones during their childhood and teenage years are more than 5 times as likely to develop a malignant brain tumor. This same study showed that people who start using a cell phone in their later years are 1.5 times as likely to develop a brain tumor as the population in general. People using household cordless phones for more than 10 years were also found to be at an increased risk.[10]

A connection between electromagnetic radiation from high-voltage power lines and childhood leukemia was shown in 1979 in a Colorado study by Dr. Nancy Wertheimer and Ed Leeper. This link was clearly evident among people who had grown up in a house surrounded by high-voltage power lines, with an especially strong

---

[8] Judith A. Westman et al., "Low Cancer Incidence Rates in Ohio Amish," *Cancer Causes Control* (2009), doi: 10.1007/SI0552-009-9435-7.

[9] Stephon Lonn et al., "Mobile Use and the Risk of Acoustic Neuroma," *Epidemiology,* 15, no. 6 (2007): 653-659.

[10] L. Hardell & M. Carlberg, Mobile Phones, Cordless Phones and the Risk for Brain Tumours," *International Journal of Oncology,* 35, no. 1, July 2009: 5-17.

incidence of leukemia among children who had spent their entire lives at one address.[11]

Based on this and similar studies, the World Health Organization (WHO) in 2002 listed power-frequency electromagnetic fields as a possible cause of childhood leukemia.[12] Then, in 2011, WHO also recognized a possible link between radio frequency electromagnetic fields and cancer.[13] These two pronouncements reflect concern over the health threats posed by electromagnetic radiation in a range of frequencies and from a wide variety of sources.

A growing body of evidence supports these health concerns. The Bio Initiative 2012 Report, compiled by epidemiologist Dr. David Carpenter and EMF expert Cindy Sage, summarizes more than 1,800 studies that investigate the effects of exposure to power lines, mis-configured electrical wiring, appliances, cordless phone systems, mobile phones, cellular antennas, transmitting utility meters, Wi-Fi, baby monitors, and other electronics. The numerous studies in this comprehensive report linked EMF exposure to everything from sleep disturbances and learning disabilities to Alzheimer's and cancer.

Even though man-made radiation is invisible, it has somehow attracted the attention of an army of scientists and researchers, resulting in a massive body of evidence to suggest that it is a very real health threat. What, then, keeps so many people from hearing the evidence and taking this threat seriously? Let's look at that next.

---

[11] Nancy Wertheimer and Ed Leeper, "Electrical Wiring Configurations and Childhood Cancer," *American Journal of Epidemiology 109,* 3, 1979: 273-284.
[12] "Electromagnetic Fields and Public Health," World Health Organization, October 2001.
[13] "IARC Classifies Radiofrequency Electromagnetic Fields as Possibly Carcinogenic to Humans," World Health Organization, May 2011.

Chapter Three

Resisting the Warnings of Science

After uncovering so much compelling evidence of the harmful effects of electromagnetic radiation on human health, I started to see the world in a whole new way. I had been around electricity for all of my life and exposed to a steadily increasing amount of electronic technology throughout my adult years. Yet, during all of this time, I had never really stopped to consider how this exposure might be impacting my health.

I'm not sure how a major health threat revealed by scientific and epidemiological research makes the leap from the world of science into the consciousness of the general public. If the threat is obvious enough, such as the sudden outbreak of a disease, this is all that it typically takes to get the public's attention. When, however, a health issue is slow to develop and its causes are cloaked in mystery, it can be difficult for people to pay much attention to the possible health dangers revealed by science, especially when they only receive those revelations in brief sound bites on the evening news.

Certainly, the health threat posed by our mounting exposure to man-made radiation is one that is especially difficult to grasp for the average person in today's high-tech world. Aside from our general ignorance of the research that points to this danger, our reactive thoughts so often prevent us from hearing, exploring, and heeding the warnings of science. Any number of faulty beliefs or notions, which seem perfectly reasonable on the surface, can effectively keep us in the dark. Let's look at some of the major ones.

I love my technology. It can't be bad for me!

Whenever we are told that something we have come to love is in some way bad for us, it is only natural that we would be quick to reject that idea. This was undoubtedly the reaction of many smokers when it was first shown that smoking could be a potential cause of emphysema and lung cancer. It is also how many people react when they are told that one of their favorite foods is unhealthy. (How could something that tastes so good be bad for me?)

In both of these cases, it is quite possible (and perhaps even probable) that an element of physical or psychological addiction is involved. Smokers come to crave their cigarettes just as food lovers may be drawn again and again to that special unhealthy food that they can't seem to live without. In both instances, the pleasure they gain in the moment from their addiction far outweighs, in their minds, any potential danger or health risk.

Electrical and electronic technology can also be addictive. We love our computers, cell phones, and other electronic devices and gadgets. They are fun to use, keep us connected to the world, and make our lives easier in so many ways. How could anything so useful and valuable be harmful as well?

This thought alone can stop us from seriously considering any health concerns that are raised related to all of the radiation that is being generated in our electrified, gadget-filled, high-tech world. And with so many technology companies selling us on the benefits of the latest emerging technology and stoking our hunger for the next new electronic wonder, it is so easy for any related health concerns to be drowned out or go unnoticed.

With electricity and electronic technology woven through the fabric of our lives, we can also feel a bit threatened when it is suggested that any resulting radiation may be harmful to our health. It is as if we are being asked to give up our cell phones and computers and go live in a cave in some remote part of the world. In reality, though, it is not necessary to go to these extremes. For the most part, we just need to take some simple precautions to safeguard our health.

When our mindset is all-or-nothing, however, it can be hard to consider that possibility. Instead, we are primed to embrace yet another faulty notion:

Electromagnetic radiation is everywhere. You can't escape it, so why try?

Indeed, we now live in a world filled with so much electromagnetic radiation that it seems almost inescapable. Our wired homes and workplaces are connected to a power grid that channels the electricity we need to heat and cool our indoor environment, light up our rooms, and power the wide range of appliances and electronic devices that have become a part of our everyday lives.

Add to this the flood of microwave/radio frequency radiation generated by all of the wireless technology in our world. A growing number of homes and businesses have wi-fi networks to allow for wireless Internet access. Our landscape is dotted with thousands of cellular towers and antennas, transmitting pulsed microwave signals to millions of cell phones. Utility companies are also adding to the mix by implementing a widespread rollout of digital transmitting utility meters.

As we are drowning in a sea of man-made radiation, it may certainly seem that we are helpless to do anything to keep from being engulfed by it all. But is that really the case?

While it may be an insurmountable task to try to change the world, there is much we can do to control our little corner of it. We can choose how we use and interact with the technology in our lives. We can find ways to minimize our exposure to electromagnetic fields. We can create safe and supportive living and working environments that still allow us to enjoy all of the benefits of electrical power and the technology that serves us so well.

Simply ignoring a potential danger that seems to be beyond your control is not the answer. When you do that, you only put yourself at greater risk. That is like walking haphazardly through a mine field when, with just a little effort, you could have first found out where the mines were located and what you needed to do to avoid them.

Of course, the most dangerous sources of man-made radiation are not set, like a land mine with a delicate trigger, to instantly explode and do us harm. The damage they enact only unfolds slowly, often imperceptibly, as we spend more and more time in the wake of their invisible, radiating fields. Being oblivious to this danger in the moment, it is easy for us to gain a false sense of security.

Surely, we would know if all of the electronics and electrical devices in our lives were causing us any harm. In the absence of any clear experiential evidence to show us otherwise, though, it is only natural that we would be led to draw the following conclusion:

All of this radiation doesn't seem to bother me. So why worry about it?

Worry is not an effective remedy for anything. But just because you have yet to notice any major ill effects of living in our electromagnetic world, that's not proof that you have no cause for concern.

Because electromagnetic stress can be quite subtle, it can do its harm without calling attention to itself, almost like an enemy spy sneaking in to sabotage the fortress of your body. Of course, your body has the ability to defend itself against this kind of assault, at least up to a point. When under acute stress, your body produces stress hormones to mount a defense and can activate your immune system to combat the onset of disease.

But if the stress persists, as is the case with ongoing exposure to harmful levels of electromagnetic radiation, your hormone and immune levels will drop well below normal. Your body will, in essence, become de-sensitized to the stress. As a result, it will be slow to activate its natural defenses, making you even more susceptible to other stressors and priming you for fatigue and illness.

Some individuals whose EMF exposure reaches a tipping point will develop Electro-hypersensitivity Syndrome, a condition in which they experience noticeable symptoms or health issues when in close contact with electromagnetic fields. The California Department of Health reported that 3% of Californians feel that they have some form of this syndrome. If everyone had this syndrome, it would be much easier for people to see electromagnetic radiation as a health concern. But since this condition only seems to affect a small percentage of the population, it is often regarded by many as an allergy, only affecting those whose unique biology makes them susceptible to it.

This, in turn, can lead everyone else to think that ongoing EMF exposure is only a health threat for an unfortunate few. Meanwhile, if you are among the "fortunate many," those who seem to be unaffected by all of this radiation, you may find yourself being worn down by the ravages of electro-stress with no clear sense of what is responsible.

Unlike those who are hypersensitive to EMFs, you may feel perfectly fine when entering or spending time in a radiation-filled environment. Sometime later, though, you may feel fatigued or experience different symptoms related to your earlier EMF exposure. But because of the time gap between your exposure and the symptoms, you simply don't connect the two.

If you had eaten some week-old stew from your refrigerator and gotten a stomach ache an hour or two later, you probably could have quickly figured out what was making you so sick. That is because you naturally link digestive issues with eating. Most likely, though, you simply don't have this type of natural mental link between EMF exposure and any related health issues that may arise. Because man-made radiation has become such a normal part of our world, you have no reason to think of it as a possible trigger for fatigue and illness.

Then, when your health starts to fade, you may simply blame it on the overall stresses of life or accept it as a natural part of the aging process. Since a gradual decline in your health and vitality can be due to a combination of different factors, it is easy for any one of these factors to blend in with the rest, even one that may be driving the decline. And if this decline is gradual enough, you may not even be aware of it from one day to the next. As a result, what you perceive as "feeling fine" today may be much less fine than you felt 5 or 10 years ago.

When you are feeling bad enough or are beset with one health issue or another, you may finally seek out a doctor or other health practitioner to fix you. If you find a doctor that you like, one who serves you well, you may then feel that you have all of the support and guidance you need to recover from what ails you. While it can certainly be reassuring to know that you have this kind of support, this may lead you to rely too much on your doctor and feel even less responsible for maintaining your own health. This, in turn, may lead you to embrace another thought:

If radiation is a major health concern, my doctor will surely let me know about it.

Good doctors make their patients' health and welfare a priority. Their focus, though, is on assessing their patients' health issues and seeing what can be done to address them. In the process, they may also offer some advice on healthy living. But typically, they only dole out this advice in small doses when they have the time and it seems appropriate.

If the health threat posed by EMF exposure was widely recognized by doctors and other health practitioners, many would undoubtedly warn their patients about it. The trouble is that most healthcare professionals do not recognize or fully understand this danger themselves. They may be better educated about health-related matters than the average person. But since, like everyone else, they are part of a world that has electromagnetic radiation as a backdrop, it is not something that typically surfaces as a concern in their thinking.

My wife Jacqueline was, in many ways, an exception to this rule. As a healthcare professional who practiced a technique called Total Body Modification (TBM), she not only recognized the negative impact of EMFs on human health but had ways of helping her patients recover from EMF stress and bring their bodies back into balance. Much of her practice, in fact, involved treating patients whose health had been compromised by different factors in their environment.

As a holistic healer, she was always learning, expanding her knowledge of health and how she could be of most help to her patients. With so much to learn, though, it was almost impossible to dive deeply into every dimension of health. She therefore tended to devote more of her attention to the subjects she was most passionate about (such as nutrition and homeopathy) and less attention to other subjects that might help to round out her health knowledge.

One such subject that was further down her list of things to explore was the nature of electromagnetic stress. She knew that man-made radiation was a health concern. She knew how to treat patients whose bodies were disrupted by exposure to electromagnetic radiation. She offered health supplements to help her patients become more resistant to electromagnetic stress and recommended different devices they might use to help harmonize that stress in their living and working environment. All of this, she had thought, was surely enough to address the issue.

But what if there was much more to staying healthy in our electromagnetic world than Jacqueline had realized? She was obviously curious about this possibility, as earlier in the final year of her life she had bought Ann Louise Gittleman's newly released book Zapped, which was a practical manual for living and working safely with our technology. I don't believe, though, that Jacqueline had ever actually read this book.

When I finally found the book Zapped on Jacqueline's desk and started reading it a month after her passing, it became increasingly clear to me how a mounting level of electromagnetic radiation had crept into our lives and escaped her attention. Over the 25+ years that Jacqueline had been in practice, steady advances in technology had dramatically changed the whole electromagnetic makeup of the world. With the growth of digital technology and wireless communication, there were more frequencies of invisible radiating signals permeating our environment than ever before.

Personal computers, laptops, cell phones, cordless phone systems, wi-fi networks, and a host of wireless devices had rolled into our world to become commonplace. Naturally, it was easy to get swept up in the excitement of all of these developments without fully considering how they might add to our level of electromagnetic stress. As a result, steps we had taken in the past to cope with this kind of stress might no longer be sufficient.

This made me wonder: could the electromagnetic environment in our home have been a major cause of our recurring health issues over the 10 years since we had moved in? We had taken so many steps to live a healthy lifestyle and create an environmentally friendly home. But could we have overlooked a subtle threat that had been robbing us of our health and keeping us from living life to the fullest? Could this invisible assailant have been what also led to Jacqueline's final illness, the one that had taken her from me forever?

It seemed that the only way for me to find out was to take what I was learning about electromagnetic radiation, evaluate the electrical environment in my home, make any changes needed to reduce and minimize my radiation exposure, and see what, if any, effect this might have on the way that I felt. So that's exactly what I did.

Chapter Four

Transforming My Environment

Armed with my new-found knowledge and understanding of electromagnetic radiation, I started looking at my home the same way that a detective would search for clues at a crime scene. I didn't have to be Sherlock Holmes, however, to discover the most glaring radiation-filled hot spot in my home—the area right around Jacqueline's computer desk chair, a chair she had sat in almost every evening for the previous 10 years.

Starting with the Electrical Hot Spot

On the floor underneath Jacqueline's desk, about a foot away from where she had placed her feet, was a wireless router, projecting its waves of RF radiation. Making matters worse, there was one cordless phone base on the desk surface to the immediate right of where she had sat and another on the work surface to the rear. Being near even one of these sources of microwave radiation for any length of time was unhealthy. But here, she had placed herself in the middle of 3 of these zappers, which was almost like sitting in the center of a big microwave oven.

I had read about different studies that found a dramatic increase in the incidence of brain tumors among people who were heavy cell phone users for 10 years or longer. Since we had also been working out of our home office for 10 years when doctors discovered a grapefruit-size tumor in Jacqueline's lower abdomen, these studies suddenly had a whole new level of significance to me. Instead, though, of holding a cell phone to her head for 2 or 3 hours a day, Jacqueline had been sitting at her computer with a wireless router underneath her desk, positioned to irradiate the lower part of her body, where the tumor was found.

Adding even more electromagnetic radiation to the mix was the jumble of electrical cords under Jacqueline's desk, a computer tower to the immediate left of her chair, a printer to the left of the computer monitor, and a large combination copying machine, scanner, and printer off to the right rear. My computer workstation was off to one side of this electronic conglomeration, so I wasn't getting nearly the level of electromagnetic exposure that Jacqueline had. Still, I could see how all of this could have been contributing to my stress symptoms and fatigue.

Wanting to reduce my radiation exposure as soon as possible, I started to take some corrective actions. I moved my computer tower farther away from where I sat. I disabled my computer wi-fi. I slid the electrical cords underneath my desk as far away as possible. I replaced my two cordless DECT phone systems with a 2-line corded landline phone.

I then surveyed the other rooms in my house and made any changes I thought would be helpful. I installed electrical filters in many of my outlets to reduce radiation surges generated by my household electrical wiring. I unplugged all of the cordless phones throughout my house. I had my electrician replace all of my lighting dimmer switches (another major cause of excess radiation) with regular light switches. I removed the television and cable box from my bedroom to create a more peaceful sleeping environment. Taking one step after another, I was determined to do whatever I could to zap-proof my home and make it the ultimate haven for health that Jacqueline and I had always wanted it to be.

After making these environmental fixes, which I did in different stages, I soon seemed to be feeling much better. At first, I wondered, though, if I was just imagining this because I expected to feel better or if, in fact, the changes I had made were having a positive effect on me. Then, one day, I had an experience that gave me the answer.

Discovering My Electromagnetic Sensitivity

The day after I disconnected my two cordless phone systems, it struck me that I hadn't erased the voice mail answering messages on them. So to handle this, I reconnected the base units of these systems and started paging through one of the instruction manuals to find the procedure for erasing this type of message. As I did this, I noticed a slight burning sensation in my chest, a feeling that grew stronger and stronger with each passing minute. When I then erased the messages and disconnected the phone bases once again, my burning sensation quickly faded away.

Obviously, the radiation from those cordless phones had been having a stressful effect on me. I had never made this connection before, since I had always simply accepted these phones as a normal part of my working environment, an environment that, for the most part, I had considered to be a healthy one. Also, during most of the time I had spent in my home office in the past, I had been so entranced by whatever was on my computer screen that I remained largely unaware of my body or how I was feeling from moment to moment.

But now, through this accidental comparison test between an environment with and without cordless phones installed, I knew that direct exposure to the phones' radio frequency radiation was bad news.   I could feel the difference.

This experience also helped me to make an important discovery about myself.   Somehow I had become at least moderately sensitive to electromagnetic radiation.   I'm sure that I had this sensitivity for some time.   I had just never drawn any connection between how I was feeling and what electrical or electronic equipment happened to be in my environment.

In a way, this was like discovering that I had a super power—the ability to sense electromagnetic fields that were undetectable to most other people.   This wasn't the kind of power that would inspire anyone to feature me as a super hero in a comic book (Radiation Detection Man?).   In fact, it might even be viewed as a weakness, similar to what Superman experienced whenever he came into close range of any kryptonite.

I soon found, though, that my electrical sensitivity was quite useful as a means of detecting any harmful radiation and thus enabling me to take steps to avoid, reduce, or eliminate my exposure to it.   In that way, my super power was a lot like the tingling sense that Spider-Man experiences whenever danger is lurking nearby.   So just maybe my electrical sensitivity could qualify me for super hero status after all!

All I knew is that after discovering my sensitivity to electromagnetic radiation, I suddenly felt empowered.   No longer did I have to go through life unnecessarily exposing myself to harmful radiation, unaware of how this invisible assailant was causing my stress levels to soar and my energy to plummet. I now had the awareness needed to create a healthy living and working environment and avoid electromagnetic hot spots whenever possible.

To identify and gauge the strength of radiation that I couldn't readily sense in my body, I also bought a detection meter that measured the strength of both electrical and magnetic fields. With my trusty meter in hand, I then went around my house and tested every electrical or electronic device. Some radiation sources, like my flat screen computer monitor and overhead incandescent lights showed a low to moderate reading. Taking my meter reading to the max, however, were such sources as cordless phone bases, digital clocks, and base of my desk lamp.

Based on what I discovered, I continued to make changes in my home and office environment, replacing high radiation devices with lower radiation ones or repositioning things to maximize my distance from the radiation source. About a year after doing all of this, I felt about 70% better than I did before. This clearly showed me that the steps I had taken were helping.

Unraveling a Mysterious Electrical Issue

While I had done a lot to improve the electrical environment in my home, I still had this deep sense that I was missing something important. Although I was minimizing the amount of time that I was spending at my computer and had taken a number of steps to lower my radiation exposure in my home office, there were times when I felt more stressed out at my computer than I felt I had any right to be. Also, in general, my overall level of stress and fatigue would rise noticeably by early afternoon, making it increasingly difficult for me to focus and accomplish anything of real value for the rest of the day.

What could be causing me to feel this way? Turning to my electrical sensitivity super power, I could only come up with one possible clue. There were two main rooms in my home that were uncarpeted, each having a tile floor. One was my kitchen; the other my home office. Whenever I stood in one of these rooms in my bare feet or stocking feet, I could feel what felt like a slight electrical charge coming up from the floor and into the soles of my feet. The longer I stood there, the stronger and more uncomfortable this sensation became.

My home was partially heated by radiant heating from the floors. That, however, relied on a network of hot water pipes under the flooring, nothing electrical. Unable to make sense of this, I finally called in my electrician to get his opinion. After evaluating the situation, he was unable to offer me any explanation for the electrical charge I was feeling in the floor. As he was unable to feel this charge himself, I also had the impression that he thought that I was a bit crazy or subject to hallucinations for thinking that an electrical issue even existed.

Convinced that I needed a second, more educated opinion about my issue, I tracked down an electrical environmental consultant named Sal La Duca to do an electrical assessment of my home. Sal brought his own highly sensitive electrical detection equipment, as well as a wealth of knowledge about electrical issues that could impact the environment in a home or office. Clearly explaining what he was discovering at each stage of his assessment, he in essence gave me a highly informative and enlightening seminar about the electrical environment in my home.

Most impressive was how quickly he figured out the cause of the electrical charge I was sensing in my kitchen and home office floors. After turning off my home's electrical power, Sal found that there was still current flowing through the pipes in my hydronic heating system. How was this possible? "Where is this current coming from?" I asked.

"What's happening here," said Sal, "is something that your electrician never stopped to consider. The electrical system feeding your home is multi-grounded, connected to other homes in the neighborhood. Current flow on the ground wire between transformers in the system will force some current to flow through the soil. Since the system ground is also your home's electrical ground, some current may flow through the soil at each home, even with the power off. Thus, apparently, the metal piping in your hydronic heating system became an additional grounding point for some of this stray current."

Mystery solved. As I never could have figured out all of this on my own, I was so glad that I had turned to an electrical environmental expert for help. Still, my next thought was, "How complicated and involved would it be to fix the problem and stop this unwanted current from radiating up through my flooring?"

Fortunately, Sal then offered me a solution that was much less involved than anything I was imagining. I simply needed to have a plumber install plastic, non-conductive tubular spacers or dielectrics in the source and return pipes of the hydronic heating system in my boiler room. This would effectively interrupt the circuit through which stray current had been passing.

What About Wiring and Electric Filters?

Sal also noticed that I had electric filters plugged into numerous electrical outlets throughout my house. I had installed these to reduce the excess radiation that can result from voltage spikes and swings in the wiring. Having done my research on these filters, I felt confident that Sal would applaud my wisdom in installing them. As it turned out, though, this simply opened the door to a deeper discussion.

"These filters," noted Sal, "are essentially capacitors, which can in fact reduce a limited range of electrical interference in your household wiring. If, however, your home has any wiring errors or the wiring is configured in certain ways, the use of these filters may be of little value. Also, since each filter is plugged into an electrical outlet, it is drawing a current. This not only adds a bit to your electric bill but could also help to create a magnetic field."

Fortunately, Sal offered me a fairly simple solution to address these concerns. All that I most likely needed was one strategically placed filter for each of the two main phases of current in my electrical system. I first needed to have an electrician see that each of the two buses or conducting bars (for these phases) at my main electrical panel was connected to a separate receptacle in my nearby double outlet. By then plugging a filter into each of two receptacles, I could effectively treat all of the circuits throughout my home.

Of course, to minimize any excess electrical interference in my wiring, he also recommended that I do whatever I could to eliminate the cause of that interference. This included replacing fluorescent lamps with incandescent or quartz halogen bulbs and eliminating my ionizing air filters, which produce both ELF radiation and radio frequency radiation. Had I not already removed my DECT cordless phone system and had an electrician eliminate my dimmer switches, these would have also been on Sal's list of offending technology to go.

Finding Ways to Further De-Stress My Office

Sal also made a couple of recommendations for improving the electrical environment in my home office. Much of the work surface in this office consisted of plywood configured in a U-shape around my late wife Jacqueline's computer desk chair. This surface was supported by metal filing cabinets at the ends, a metal student desk at the base of the U (and to the immediate right of where Jacqueline had sat), and metal support legs at other spots where needed.

After surveying this office set-up, Sal quickly pointed out an issue that had been invisible to me. "Your metal desk and leg supports," said Sal, "are a real problem here. Being so close to your computer equipment and the jumble of electrical cords on the floor, all of this metal is conducting and amplifying the nearby electrical fields. To fix this, you need to ditch these metal supports and replace them with wooden legs or tables."

As Jacqueline's computer desk chair was right in the middle of this metal support system, it became clear to me that she had been sitting in an even more electrically toxic environment than I had imagined. My computer desk, made of wood, was off to one side and farther away from all of this metal, giving me some distance from this high-radiation zone. Still, being as electrically sensitive as I was,

I could see how I might be affected by this metal leg support system as well.

Sal also noticed that I had an earthing/grounding mat underneath my computer desk.   This was a small rectangular mat that attached with a cord to the grounding port in the electrical outlet behind my desk. I had read that sitting with my feet on this kind of mat was a good way to keep myself grounded, reduce inflammation, and neutralize the ongoing negative effects of exposure to electromagnetic radiation.

Feeling quite proud of how smart I was for using this kind of mat, I fully expected Sal to praise me for this. Surprisingly, though, he started to shake his head back and forth in disapproval. "While you're revamping your office," he said, "you may also want to eliminate that grounding mat.   By sitting with your feet on that mat in such an electrically charged environment, you are turning your body into an antenna or human lightning rod."

It seemed that in trying to protect myself from excess radiation, I had been actually making the problem worse! As I had been sitting so close to the metal desk supports, which had also been acting as electrical antennas, I could see why I was still feeling stressed in my office, even after taking so many other steps to reduce my radiation exposure. Once again, I felt so glad that I had turned to an electrical environmental expert for help.

A Finishing Touch for a Low-Stress Bedroom

One other important room that I asked Sal about was my bedroom. I had a wooden bed frame and slept on a latex rubber mattress, so I didn't have to worry about the close contact I would have with conductive metal had I had a metal bed frame and wire spring mattress. I had also removed the television, cable box, video recorder, and cordless phone that had been in our bedroom for many years. Eliminating all of these electronics had almost immediately made this room a more peaceful and harmonious place to rest and recharge. Still, I wondered if there might be something else I could do to improve this sleeping environment even more.

Sure enough, Sal had an idea for me. As the head of my bed was against a wall that had two electrical outlets and wiring feeding them, he noted that this was creating an electrical field that I was exposed to as I slept. To eliminate this field, he suggested that I have my electrician create a switched circuit in my bedroom so that the electricity in the walls closest to me could be turned off at night.

Yes, the electrical field coming from the wiring in my bedroom walls may have been quite subtle. But didn't I want my sleeping environment to be as stress-free as possible? My body was already exposed to plenty of electromagnetic stress throughout the day without adding to it each night as I slept. To allow myself to fully recover from the stresses of the day, it was clear that I needed to do everything possible to make my bedroom the most supportive place for this restorative magic to happen.

Implementing My EMF Consultant's Advice

Impressed with all that I had learned from Sal, I proceeded to implement his recommendations for reducing the levels of electromagnetic radiation in my home. I first had a plumber perform Sal's suggested fix for eliminating the electrical charge that had been coming from the pipes underneath my flooring. Afterwards, I stood on both my kitchen floor and home office floor in my bare feet and was happy to discover that the electrical charge was gone. The fix had worked!

On a side note, the plumber who performed the above fix was actually the second one I had contacted about doing this job. The first one I spoke to found it so unbelievable that this procedure would fix my problem that he refused to do it. This experience, along with my previous interaction with an electrician who, in essence, told me that my electrical problem wasn't possible, showed me that certain electrical environmental issues are beyond the understanding of contractors who may otherwise seem to be quite qualified and reputable.

A week or two later, I brought in an electrician to do the electrical work Sal had recommended. I first had my electrician perform a little electrical bypass surgery on my two-receptacle outlet at my main electric panel. This resulted in having each receptacle connected to a separate bus or conducting bar, one for each of the two main phases of current in my electrical system. I then plugged an electric filter into each of these receptacles and removed the other filters from the outlets throughout my house.

Using a micro-surge testing meter, I then went through my home to test my household outlets. Most every reading was quite low and well within the "safe" range. One noticeable exception, which showed an extremely high reading, was an outlet that had a photo-catalytic air purifier plugged into it. As this purifier contained a fluorescent bulb and generated both ELF and radio frequency radiation, I could see why it was near the top of Sal's hit list for removal. And now I had some sky high numbers to show me how much interference it was creating on my home's electrical wiring.

I also had my electrician create a switched electrical circuit in my bedroom. After then being able to turn off the electricity in the wiring near my bed night, I seemed to be sleeping more peacefully than ever. Finally, my bedroom truly was a haven for rest and rejuvenation.

My one remaining major project was to address the situation in my home office. This involved replacing the metal desk and legs supporting the plywood work surface in our "electrical corner" with 3 small wooden tables. This eliminated the excess electrical field conductors that had existed when so much metal had been in the environment.

After making this change, I felt much better when working at my computer. Suddenly, I was able to work comfortably for much longer periods of time than I had ever remembered being able to do since moving into the house. I still didn't want to push myself and try to set any endurance records for time spent in front of a computer. But it was great to be able to sit at my workstation long enough to accomplish a nice chunk of work without feeling deflated or stressed out as I was just getting started.

As I had already taken so many other steps to reduce my electrical field exposure in my home office, it seemed that the elimination of so much metal just might be the final major missing piece to lowering my electrical stress and making this a place in which I could work productively.

What a Difference!

As of this writing, it has now been over a year since I made all of these environmental changes in my home. Since I first moved into this house 14 years ago, this has been the first year that my stress levels have not been on a rollercoaster ride of ups and downs, the first year in which my mysterious stress syndrome hasn't surfaced to slow me down or immobilize me every few months or so, the first year in which I've been able to embrace the belief that I can sustain the energy needed to live a full, productive life.

I know that there is a lot of controversy surrounding the potential health hazards of electromagnetic radiation and, in particular, the seemingly harmless non-ionizing radiation produced by cell phones, wi-fi networks, and other wireless electronic devices. There have been many studies conducted to prove the existence of these health hazards and many others to cast doubt upon them.

I, however, didn't need scientists and researchers to conduct an exhaustive study to convince me of the harmful effects of the man-made radiation that is so widespread in today's world. My experience, and that of my late wife Jacqueline, provided me with all of the proof that I needed.

What all did I learn from my journey of discovery? I learned how dangerous electromagnetic radiation can be— even though this danger or its ill effects may be undetectable in the moment. I discovered how ongoing exposure to high levels of man-made radiation can promote ill health and fatigue in the short run and become life-threatening in the long run. I learned that it is eminently possible to minimize these health risks by becoming aware of your environment and taking steps to minimize your radiation exposure in your daily life.

My hope is that my story has opened up this same path of enlightenment to you so that you too can live the full, vital, productive life that you were put on this earth to live. To guide you down this path, I share with you, in the next chapter, some steps you can take to create a healthier living and working environment and minimize the hidden dangers of living in this age of high technology.

Chapter Five

Creating a Safe Place
To Live and Work

From reading my story, you learned the steps I took to reduce my exposure to electromagnetic stress, create a healthier living and working environment, and reclaim my health and vitality. So that you can easily do the same, here are some basic guidelines for you to follow:

Create a Low-EMF Living Environment

1. Live as far away as possible from high-voltage power lines, transformers, and cell phone antennas.

2. Use energy-efficient appliances.

3. Avoid cordless phone systems, particularly DECT versions, which emit microwave radiation even when not in use. Instead, use traditional corded landline phones.

4. Don't use microwave ovens. Or if you do, stand clear of them when they are in use.

5. Place high-EMF appliances, such as refrigerators and cathode ray tube televisions, against outer walls. Positioned against interior walls, they can be sending high levels of radiation into the next room.

6. Do not use a ceiling fan in a room below a bedroom or other room where people spend a lot of time.

7. If at all possible, locate your primary living and sleeping areas as far away as possible from any utility "smart meters." Or better yet, if you can, opt out of any initiative by your utility company to install smart meters outside your home.

8. Replace bulky cathode ray tube televisions with models having LCD screens, which have much lower electrical fields. (Note: many large-screen TVs can create high-frequency fields throughout a room.)

9. Position your chairs, sofas or couches at least 6-7 feet away from your television. The greater the distance, the better.

10. Stay clear of electrical wires, power cords, and surge protectors, which all project electric fields.

11. To reduce the electrical surges and harmonics on your household wiring, install electrical filters in outlets near your electrical panel, one for each of your two main electrical lines. (To do this, you may first need to have an electrician see that each main line is connected to a nearby outlet.)

12. Eliminate or disable wi-fi and use Ethernet cables to connect with the Internet. If you can't bring yourself to do this, keep your wireless router as far away as possible from where you spend most of your time. Also, keep your wi-fi router turned off when not needed and definitely at night.

De-Stress Your Bedroom

Your bedroom is the place for you to rest and recover from the stresses of your day. So that you can sleep deeply and peacefully each night and your body is best able to work its restorative magic, do whatever you can to minimize the EMFs in this place of rest. Here is how:

1. Don't use an electric blanket or heated water bed.

2. Switch from an electric alarm clock to a battery-powered one.

3. Never sleep near a cell phone or cordless DECT phone that is turned on or charging.

4. Optimally, remove all electronic devices from your bedroom. If you do have any such devices in your bedroom, make sure that they are unplugged while you sleep. (Digital TVs, for instance, emit radiation even when they are turned off but still plugged in.)

5. If you have wi-fi in your home, turn it off at night.

6. Select a bed with a wooden frame and a latex rubber foam mattress, avoiding wire spring mattresses.

7. Have an electrician connect the electrical circuit in your bedroom to a switch, so that the current running through the wiring in your bedroom walls can be turned off at night. (Or alternatively, you might reduce your EMF exposure by moving your bed at least several inches from any wall.)

Make Smart Choices for Lighting

Some artificial light sources will generate stronger electromagnetic fields than others. Certain light fixture switches can also create unhealthy levels of radiation. Here are some guidelines to help you make the best choices:

1. Light Bulbs and Lamps to Avoid

   a) Fluorescent lights, both the long rod and compact curly-shaped versions (CFL's, which might more aptly stand for Chronic Fatigue Lights). They generate unhealthy levels of radiation, create interference on your household wiring, and contain mercury, which can pose a health hazard if the bulb were to break.

   b) LED lamps fed off of 120 VAC. These have a switching power supply that produces harmonics or interference that is similar to or worse than that of compact fluorescent bulbs (CFLs).

   c) Low-voltage halogen lighting products.

2. Preferred Light Bulbs and Lamps

   a) Line-voltage (120 V) halogen lamps

   b) Conventional or daylight incandescent bulbs

3. Use light fixture cords with shielded wiring. (The electric field range for a table lamp and unshielded cord will span five feet or more.)

4. Replace dimmer switches with regular switches. Dimmers produce strong bands of added radiation.

5. Have an electrician rewire lights controlled by multiple switches so that only one switch is connected. Multiple switches, when improperly installed, can create magnetic fields.

6. If a light flickers, get an electrician to replace its switch and check for a loose connection.

7. When natural daylight streaming in through windows is sufficient to meet your lighting needs, keep artificial lights turned off.

Make Your Office a Safer Place to Work

Naturally, your office or home office is a room that typically contains a lot of electronic equipment. While it is probably not possible to make this a radiation-free zone, here are some guidelines to help you minimize your EMF exposure and safeguard your health.

1. Keep power cords organized and as far away from your feet as possible. (Overlapping cords can result in increased electrical field emissions.) Use shielded power cords to reduce your radiation exposure.

2. Eliminate or disable wi-fi and use Ethernet cables to connect with the Internet.

3. If you have wi-fi (not recommended), keep your wireless router as far away from your workstation as possible. Also, keep your wireless function turned off when not needed.

4. If you have a wireless keyboard and/or mouse, replace it with a corded version.

5. Keep your computer hard drive at least a few feet away from you.

6. When you have no immediate need for a nearby piece of office equipment (such as a printer or paper shredder), keep it turned off and/or unplugged.

7. Replace metal desks with wooden ones.

8. Avoid having office equipment all around you.

9. Replace cordless DECT phone systems with corded landlines.

Detect and Measure EMFs

Following the EMF safety guidelines in this chapter will help you minimize your exposure to electromagnetic fields. It can also be helpful, though, to have a means of detecting and measuring EMFs. This will allow you to identify radiation hot spots, evaluate the electromagnetic punch packed by the appliances and devices that you currently use, and help you to choose the safest electronics to buy.

A crude device for detecting EMFs is an AM transistor radio with an analog dial. By tuning the dial to a point where you have no reception from any station, you can use the level of static that you hear as an audible indicator of the strength of any nearby EMFs. The closer you hold the radio to any EMF-producing device, the louder or more pronounced the static will become. When holding your radio next to an EMF source generating an extra-high level of radiation, such as digital clock or cordless phone base, you will most likely hear the static noise turn into a sharp, loud buzz.

To measure EMF levels, you can buy different EMF meters that measure electric, magnetic, and radio frequency fields. A Gauss meter, for instance, measures the strength of magnetic fields, expressed as gauss or tesla. Basic guidelines for safe exposure are readings of no more than 2 to 3 mG. Most EMF experts, though, recommend that you look for a reading of 1 mG or lower to measure a safe distance between you and an EMF source such as a television or computer monitor.

Some EMF meters detect and measure the different major types of fields. Others are tailored to measuring one specific type of field. To investigate the different types of EMF meters available, visit the web sites of the suppliers listed at the end of this book.

Get Expert Help

A licensed electrician can help you reduce the amount of electromagnetic radiation in your home or office by fixing loose wiring, replacing dimmer switches with regular light switches, rewiring lights controlled by multiple switches so that only one is connected, and setting up a switched electrical circuit in your bedroom so the electric in the walls near your bed can be easily switched off at night.

To uncover and resolve hidden electrical issues creating harmful levels of electromagnetic radiation, however, you need a professional with more specialized knowledge, an electrical environmental consultant, sometimes referred to as an EMF mitigator or biological building inspector. To locate one of these experts in your area, contact the International Institute for Building-Biology and Ecology at 1-866-960-0333 or search the listing on the IBE web site at http://hbelc.org/findexpert/enviroconsult.

Protective Shields and Devices

A wide range of protective products have been developed to help shield people from the assault of electromagnetic radiation, reduce radiation levels, or neutralize the negative effects of EMFs. These include such items as protective cases and neutralizing patches for cell phones, personal protection pendants, shielding clothing, fabrics, paints, and plastics, as well as devices designed to help neutralize electromagnetic fields in a room. Reported benefits of using these types of products have included: decreased fatigue, greater energy, an improved ability to focus and concentrate, more restful sleep at night, and better overall health.

While it may seem great to have so much technology to protect us from our technology, these protective health and safety aids may not be sufficient to fully protect ourselves in this electromagnetic age. A particular protective shield may not be effective in safeguarding you from all types of radiation. A device that works well in situation may not work so well in another. It can certainly be worthwhile to explore what all you can do to protect yourself and what works for you. (See the resource section at the end of this book.) Just keep in mind that protective shields and devices may not provide the total answer.

Most important are the steps you take to minimize your exposure to electromagnetic radiation and use your electrical and electronic technology as intelligently and safely as possible. This chapter offers you many specific guidelines for doing this. It's now up to you to take action. Wondering where to start? Let's look at a few high-priority areas for you to focus on first.

Quick-Start Action Steps

This chapter contains many action steps you can take to reduce the level of electromagnetic radiation in your home and office. If you are like most people with a long list of things to do, though, you might be tempted to put all of this aside and do nothing—or put off taking any action until much later. To simplify matters and prime you for immediate action, let me share with you what I feel are the three most important matters you need to address first.

1. **Replace fluorescent lighting and lamps with incandescent bulbs or line-voltage halogen lamps.** Both compact and traditional fluorescent bulbs generate unhealthy levels of radiation and create interference on your household wiring.

2. **Remove the major sources of microwave radiation from your home and office.** This includes: a) replacing any DECT cordless phone system with corded landline phones and b) disabling your computer WiFi and instead using an Ethernet cable for Internet access.

3. **Eliminate major sources of electromagnetic radiation from your bedroom.** Televisions, video recorders, cable boxes, cordless phones, computers, electronic gaming systems—all can add harmful electromagnetic stress to your sleeping environment and detract from the quality of your sleep. Even when most digital electronics are turned off, they are still emitting radiation. So clear out these electronic assailants as soon as possible.

By simply addressing these 3 quick-start action items, you may very well eliminate most of the most harmful radiation you are now exposed to every day. You can then tackle, one step at a time, the other items from the different lists in this chapter. Get started today and lay the foundation for a longer, healthier, and more energetic life.

Chapter Six

Safeguarding
Your Personal Space

You now know some steps you can take to minimize your exposure to harmful levels of man-made radiation in your home and office. These steps require some effort. But once you have taken them, you can feel good about having created a healthier space in the places where you spend most of your time.

There is, however, a place that warrants even more of your attention, a place where you spend all of your time. This is your personal space, the space immediately surrounding your body, the space you take with you wherever you go.

Do you know how uncomfortable you feel when someone enters your personal space and stands so close to you that you can feel his breath on your face as he speaks? If this is a slightly annoying person, you could probably put up with him if he stood a few feet away. But when he is right in your face (and your space), it is simply too much.

When a strong shot of electromagnetic radiation enters your personal space, the effect is much the same. You may not be aware that your space has been invaded. But your body knows. Rather than shouting "Not so close," though, it can react in a number of defensive ways.

It may release stress hormones to raise its defenses. It may become inflamed, and not merely annoyed, by the intrusion. It may even buckle from a blow that weakens its ability to protect itself from this and other stresses in your life. In the short run, this can wear you down, chipping away at your physical and mental edge. In the long run, this blow, and others like it, can set the stage for chronic illness and disease.

What determines the overall impact of this type of assault is how directly, powerfully, and often you are hit. The closer you are to a harmful source of radiation and the more time you spend with this assailant in your personal space, the more severely you will be affected.

When a champion prize fighter moves in close and pummels his opponent with one sharp blow after another to the head and body, the effect can be devastating. To keep this from happening to them, professional boxers know that they must be ready to put up their guard and step back out of the striking range of their opponent. In short, they must protect their personal space or face the painful consequences.

To safeguard your health and ensure your survival in today's high-tech world, you must be just as vigilant. In the electromagnetic boxing ring of life, your opponents, so to speak, are all of the sources of man-made radiation that you encounter. What makes it so easy to drop your guard and let these opponents enter your personal space, however, is that they don't seem like opponents at all. In fact, they appear to be friends and allies.

Your electrical and electronic devices, after all, were designed to serve you, to make your life easier, to boost your productivity, to provide you with sources of entertainment, to enable you to easily connect and communicate with friends, family, colleagues, and business contacts. How could you even think of devices that do so much for you as being opponents?

When getting too close to you, though, even your strongest allies can step on your toes, bump into you to throw you off balance, and unintentionally hurt you. So whether you are dealing with a friend or foe, you still need to stay alert and take whatever steps are needed to protect your personal space. And the easiest and most significant one you can take may simply be a step back.

Let's say that, for some strange reason, you have a masochistic streak in you and are looking for a way to inflict as much punishment on your body as possible. Using what science has shown us about the dangers of electromagnetic fields, how might you do this?

A most effective method would be to bring a harmful source of electromagnetic radiation as close as possible to your body and vital organs and keep it there as long as you could. If you could also find a way to increase the intensity of the radiation, even better. This would not only maximize the impact of each electromagnetic punch but would keep the punches coming to steadily wear down your body without giving it time to recover. Sound like a plan?

Recognizing that masochism is highly over-rated and detrimental to your long-term health, you would never want to make this plan an ongoing part of your life. It is quite possible, though, that without realizing it, this is something that you may already be doing. This, in fact, is a common behavior pattern of thousands, if not millions, of cell phone users today.

Think about it. When you use a cell phone by pressing it tightly against your ear, you are sending a straight shot of RF/microwave radiation into your brain. If you are calling from within a car, that shot is even stronger, since your phone must work extra hard to make a connection. This also gives any other passengers a second-hand blast.

When your cell phone is turned on, even when not in use, it is still sending and receiving regular signals to stay connected to a network of cell phone antennas. If you have this activated phone clipped to your belt or carry it in one of your pants pockets, you are directly exposing your reproductive organs to these pulses of radiation. If you carry this phone in your shirt pocket or the breast pocket of your jacket, your heart and other surrounding organs are taking the hit.

If you take your switched-on cell phone to bed with you, either tucked under your pillow or setting on your night stand, you have a little more separation from it. Still, its radiation is entering your personal space and stressing your body at a time when your body needs to rest undisturbed so that it can fully recover from the many stresses of your life. And if your nearby phone is also plugged in and charging as you sleep, that only strengthens its electromagnetic punch.

What exactly is the impact of each punch or the barrage of punches that you endure? Again, that depends largely on how close you are to your radiating phone and how much time you spend close to it. For an adult talking on a cell phone held to the ear, scientists have found that the radiation penetrates about 2 inches into the brain. For children, whose skulls are thinner and brain tissue more conductive, the penetration is even deeper.

What is noteworthy, though, is how much the impact of any offending radiation can be reduced with just a little distance. When you hold a cell phone 2 inches from your head or body, the strength of the signal hitting you is only a quarter of what it is when you hold the phone right next to you. And at 4 inches, it is only 1/16 as strong. Thus, by simply using your speakerphone function to keep the phone away from your head and carrying your switched-on phone in your purse or briefcase (rather than in direct contact with your body), you can dramatically reduce your radiation exposure.

To avoid an ongoing flurry of electromagnetic punches and protect yourself further, there are some equally simple steps you can take. You can start by keeping your cell phone calls short or simply texting when you want to communicate a brief message. When you are out and it is highly unlikely that you will be receiving any important calls, you can keep your cell phone turned off and just check your messages periodically.

Unless you are an emergency responder or in a profession or situation in which it is vitally important that people have minute-to-minute access to you, there is no real need to have your cell phone turned on and invading your personal space throughout the day. At the least, you can keep your phone turned off during blocks of time when you know that you don't want to be disturbed. That way, you can reduce both your EMF exposure and the stress of being interrupted.

One of your top health priorities is getting a good night's sleep. If you're like most people, the overnight period is when you are least likely to receive any type of phone call. So is sleeping near a turned-on cell phone all night really worth all of the steady electromagnetic stress this would place on your body? And who would you want to receive a call from at 3 a.m. anyway?

If you are a heavy cell phone user (or feel that your phone has almost become a part of you, at your side 24 hour a day), taking some simple steps to protect your personal space and change your relationship with your phone may be the most significant thing you can do to reduce your overall radiation exposure. Even better, the greater awareness you develop from using your phone more consciously and safely can extend throughout your life. You will then find yourself naturally and automatically applying the same safety principles you have mastered in using your cell phone to safeguard your personal space and health when interacting with other electrical and electronic technology in your world.

You will then go from being an unknowing victim, unaware of how the electromagnetic forces around you are assaulting your body, to being a conscious guardian of your health, aware of what you must do to protect your personal space while still reaping and enjoying the benefits of this technological age.

Guidelines for Safer Cell Phone Use

1. Keep cell phone conversations short and only use your cell phone when absolutely necessary.

2. Avoid holding a cell phone against your ear, which sends microwaves directly into your brain. Use your speaker phone function or text to maintain some distance between you and your phone.

3. Do not use a cordless (Bluetooth) earpiece, which places a radio next to your head. Air tube headsets are safer, but you still need to keep the phone itself as far away from you as possible when in use.

4. Never carry a turned-on cell phone in a shirt or pants pocket, inside a bra, or clipped to a belt. This exposes your vital organs to regular pulses of microwave radiation.

5. Avoid using a mobile phone in cars, busses, elevators, airplanes, trains, and subways, since this makes your phone increase its radiation output and exposes anyone nearby to EMFs.

6. Minimize your use of a cell phone in any place where the antenna signal is weak and reception is poor. In such areas, your phone must increase its radiation output to connect with the relay antenna.

7. Avoid using cell phones or electronic tablets to send or receive pictures or movies, since this type of data requires more bandwidth and generates higher levels of radiation.

Tips for Children, Teens, and Pregnant Women

Young and developing children are especially vulnerable to the harmful effects of electromagnetic radiation. As they grow, their cells are rapidly dividing and even more susceptible to damage from EMF stress than the cells of an adult. Because a child's skull is also thinner, it offers less protection for the brain, making a young child's brain especially vulnerable to cell phone radiation.

Here are some steps to protect your child from the start:

1. If you are an expectant mother, limit your use of cell phones or household cordless phones and avoid other major sources of radiation as well. If you must use a cell phone in an emergency, keep it away from your abdomen.

2. Never use a cell phone near a baby's head.

3. Avoid using a wireless baby monitor in an infant's bedroom. If using a wired version, keep it several feet away from your baby's crib.

4. Position an infant's crib away from walls containing electrical wiring, as well as other major sources of electromagnetic fields.

5. Clear your young child's or teenager's bedroom of electronic equipment or find a way to ensure that any such device is unplugged at night. Cell phones should also be turned off before bedtime. Getting quality, stress-free sleep is vital to the healthy growth and development of children.

6. Do not buy cell phones for pre-schoolers or let them use your cell phones as toys. Delay, as long as possible, buying cell phones for school-age children.

7. Encourage your children and teens to limit their cell phone use and teach them how to use and carry their phones safely.

8. Stress to your children that they should not use a laptop computer on their laps, as this direct contact can expose their reproductive organs to excess heat, moderate to high EMFs (if the unit is plugged into a wall outlet or other power source), and microwave transmissions (if the Wi-Fi card is enabled). Set a good example by keeping your laptop computer or electronic tablet off of your lap when in use. (From a safety standpoint, "laptop" is probably the worst name ever given to an electronic device.)

Chapter Seven

Surviving and Thriving In a Wi-Fi World

The truth is that protecting yourself from the assault of electromagnetic radiation is not simply like what a professional fighter must do to defend himself against the blows of a single opponent in the boxing ring. It is quite often like being in the ring with many opponents, trying to fend off the punches coming at you from all sides.

In your life, the opponents swinging at you are the different sources of electromagnetic radiation in your environment. In your kitchen, these might include your refrigerator, electric stove, microwave oven, toaster, and any number of other electrical devices and appliances. In your office, these might include your computer, router, printer, lamps, telephone equipment and all of the cords supplying power to these devices.

Fortunately, you're not necessarily walking into an ambush when you enter one of these rooms. By simply following the safety guidelines in the previous chapter, you can keep your radiation exposure and its effect on you to a minimum. To those guidelines, though, I would add another: Whenever possible, avoid exposing yourself to multiple sources of radiation at the same time.

You wouldn't, for example, want to peer through the window of a turned-on microwave oven as you talk on your cell phone and boil water in a nearby electric kettle, effectively giving yourself a multi-source radiation shower.

Or if you are working at your desktop computer and it is near a printer or copying machine, why not keep those nearby machines turned off until you actually need to use them? Why needlessly add to the radiation level in the room when you will be sitting there for awhile?

Back when I started working as a full-time marketing writer, I had two major sources of electromagnetic radiation ganging up on me—my computer and the overhead fluorescent lights. But then, after I had worked at this job for a few years as an unknowing victim of this double-teaming effect, I started keeping the overhead fluorescents turned off and instead used a lamp with a much less stressful incandescent bulb. After making this switch, I felt better almost immediately. I only wished that I had had the sense to do this much sooner.

Unfortunately, when my wife Jacqueline and I set up our joint home office years later, neither of us had the level of awareness needed to consider how the harmful effects of electromagnetic radiation could be multiplied by having so much of our office equipment concentrated near the areas where we worked. Sadly, when Jacqueline sat at her computer workstation, she endured electromagnetic punches from all sides. She was, after all, surrounded by computer equipment, had a jumble of electrical cords and a wireless router a foot or so away from her on the floor, and had two cordless phone bases on nearby work surfaces.

She might have been able to withstand the repeated assaults of one or two of these sources of radiation. Together, though, they were simply too much for her. While her vast knowledge of healthcare enabled her to bounce back time and again from her ongoing series of health issues, she was, in the long run, no match for the invisible electromagnetic forces that surrounded her.

Only rarely did Jacqueline and I use a cell phone. Yet throughout our home was a cordless phone system that generated the same type of microwave radiation that frequent cell phone users are blasted with all the time. Whenever we used one of these home phones or were simply near one for any length of time, our personal space was invaded. As our home office contained two of these phones, along with a radiating wireless router, you might say that whenever we spent any time in this room, we had opened ourselves to a full-scale attack.

As Jacqueline sat close to these zappers, most often for an hour or two in the evening, she took the more direct hits at a time when she was already worn down by the stresses of her day. Then, when she finally went to bed for the night, a time when ideally her body should have a chance to fully rest and rejuvenate itself, the hits kept coming. Just two feet away on her nightstand was a satellite phone base, generating pulses of radiation to continue to invade her personal space and assault her body as she slept.

***

Each of us has a unique history of exposure to different forms of electromagnetic energies. Unless you live on a remote island separated from the technologies of modern life, you have your own unique series of encounters each day with various frequencies of man-made radiation. Sometimes the radiation from a few different sources will be coming at you all at once. Other times, the radiation from only one significant source may be invading your personal space. Yet other times, if you can manage to get away from it all, you may be able to take a refreshing break from the stresses of our electromagnetic world.

What's important to consider is that the overall impact of the various electromagnetic stresses in your life is cumulative. The longer and more often that your personal space is invaded by electromagnetic radiation, the greater the hit your health can take. Any one brief exposure may seem inconsequential. (So what if I get a short blast of radiation when drying my hair with an electric hair dryer?) But the cumulative effect of ongoing exposures may be more than your body can handle.

In the past, in the early decades after the world became electrified, this wasn't so much of an issue. The sources of man-made radiation were relatively few and the average person's close interaction with electrical or electronic technology was much less frequent. People's lives were aided or enriched by electrical technology without it being a major source of ongoing stress.

Today this is no longer the case. Technology has become woven into the fabric of our lives. It is filling our homes, schools, and workplaces with waves of electromagnetic radiation. Around the clock, it is at our sides and invading our personal space, where it can do the most harm.

Heralded and applauded as the most life-changing technological breakthroughs are the ones that seem to pose the greatest threats to our health. These include the digital and wireless technologies that enable us to harness the power of radio waves to make and receive calls almost anywhere with our portable communication devices, to talk on home and office phones that are free from the confinement of a cord, to easily access the Internet, with no need for a cable connection, using our laptop computers, electronic tablets, and other mobile devices. We also have wireless games, speakers, headsets, and earpieces.

New applications of wireless technology continue to emerge, only adding to the amount of electromagnetic stress in our lives. Utility companies are replacing old analog electric meters with digital radiating "smart meters" to more easily track power usage as they pump pulses of radio waves into people's homes. Wireless security systems offer an unhealthy dose of radiation as part of the "security" package. In addition to radiating GPS systems, some automobile manufacturers are also installing wi-fi capability in their cars as a bonus feature. (Who really needs another source of stress as a bonus?)

All of this advancing technology in our world certainly has its advantages. It's just that if we are not smart, careful, and judicious in how we use our technology, those advantages can be outweighed by the costs of mounting stress, sagging energy, and failing health. When that happens, we end up sacrificing our ability to live life to the fullest and becoming a slave to the technology that was designed to serve us.

To maintain our balance, we don't need to totally abandon the innovations of our high-tech age. We simply need to make our health a priority and do whatever we can to live safely in our modern world. This can be easy to do and just as easy not to do. It all depends on your ability to awaken from the technology trance of our times and your willingness to take some simple steps that can make all the difference.

In this book, I've done my best to provide you with the needed wake-up call. I've also outlined many steps you can take to survive and thrive in this wi-fi world gone wild. The rest is up to you.

To simplify matters, there are really only 3 major steps you need to take:

1. **Create a living environment that minimizes your exposure to electromagnetic fields.** Most important, make your bedroom an electronics-free zone, a nightly retreat from electro-stress.

2. **Create an office or workplace that minimizes your exposure to electromagnetic fields.**

3. **Safeguard your personal space by using your cell phone and personal electronic devices sensibly and being aware of how you interact with all of the technology in your life.**

Granted, the first two steps above, which involve reshaping your environment, may be somewhat involved and require you to bring in some outside help to implement them. This, though, is an investment of time and effort that can pay dividends for years to come.

The third step—safeguarding your personal space—is really a habit, one that you can start cultivating today by mastering the basics of using and carrying your cell phone safely.

Once you have these three elements in place, you will be set. You will have created a home and workplace designed to minimize your levels of electromagnetic stress and support your overall well-being. Equally, if not more important, you will know how to function in this brave, new, ever-changing world. You will know how to make the most of the technology that serves you best, while maintaining the vitality needed to live a long, full, rich, productive, and happy life.

Conclusion

Playing with Fire

When early man first learned how to harness the power of fire to stay warm, cook food, and light up the darkness, this was a great boon to his life. He also found, though, that if he got too close to that fire, he would get burned. And if he let that fire rage out of control, it could put his life at risk and destroy everything around him.

In today's world, we are playing with a different kind of fire. Through rapid advances in technology, we now have access to an abundance of electrical and electronic devices that have made our lives easier in so many ways. Many of these technological advances, however, pose an invisible threat that may be as dangerous as a run-away wildfire.

In a way, the health threat posed by man-made radiation may be even more dangerous than fire. Because radiation is invisible, we can't see, in the moment, how it is doing us any harm. Also, since the negative impact of radiation on our health can take months or years to surface in a noticeable way, it can remain unclear as to whether or not ongoing radiation exposure is even a major concern.

There's an old saying that goes "What you can't see won't hurt you." Today, this is one notion that we can ill afford to embrace. Now, more than ever, what we can't see is hurting us and will continue to hurt us as long as we remain blind to the hidden dangers of our high-tech age.

The most powerful weapon we have for fighting the invisible wildfire of man-made radiation is awareness.

While we may not be able to easily detect our assailant, we can become aware of where it is coming from. Armed with this awareness, we can then take steps to safeguard our health, to minimize our exposure to the most harmful sources of radiation, to create healthier homes and workplaces, and to use our technology more intelligently and safely—all while still being able to reap the benefits of the conveniences and innovations of our modern world.

It took me many years to awaken to the dangers of living in this electromagnetic age, years in which I often felt only half-alive. If it has taken you an hour or so to read this book, your awakening has thankfully been much faster. Now that you are awake, take what you have learned here to transform your life for the better. As I can attest, making some simple shifts in your habits and living environment can be life-changing.

Get started today and soon you will discover how much more alive you can feel once you have tamed the invisible wildfire of man-made radiation and increasingly have the good sense to simply unplug.

Closing Questions

Priming Yourself for Action

My hope is that this book has awakened you to the dangers of the ever-increasing amount of man-made radiation in our modern world and motivated you to take some simple steps to safeguard your health so that you can live your life to the fullest.

Of course, this book is only of real value if you actually apply the advice that it contains. I've done my best along the way to condense my advice into clear, simple steps that you can readily put into action. As a reader, though, your focus so far has been on simply digesting the ideas in this book and perhaps considering how they might be useful and relevant to your life.

To prime you for action, I will now pose some questions to help you quickly benefit from what you have learned. The questions themselves contain no real magic. The magic can be found in your answers and the actions you take as a result.

Start by taking a moment to write out your answer to the first question. You will then be ready to easily answer the other questions and spring into action. Taking that first small step today will set you in motion and make it even easier to take the second one and the one after that. As the impact of your actions continues to build, you will soon be feeling better and better, perhaps more vibrant and alive than you have in years.

Ready for that to happen? It all starts with answering Question #1.

Question #1

If you could double your energy by taking the simple steps outlined in this book, what all would that enable you to do?

(List 5-10 possibilities.)

Question #2

What is the next smallest step you will take today to reduce your ongoing exposure to electromagnetic radiation?

(Chapters 5 and 6 are chock-full of possibilities.)

Question #3

What electrical or electronic device in your bedroom will you unplug and/or remove today so that you can sleep more deeply and rejuvenate yourself more fully tonight?

(And if you are serious about getting a good night's sleep, maybe there is more than one device you'd like to unplug.)

Question #4

What are the 3 steps you will take this week to reduce the level of electromagnetic radiation in your home or office?

(Chapter 5 gives you plenty of ideas—and your list of three might even include the steps you identified in answering the previous two questions.)

Question #5

What electrical issues in your home or office will require you to enlist the help of a professional to address?

(Anything from fixing flickering lights and wiring problems to replacing dimmer switches with regular switches and creating a switched circuit in your bedroom so you can turn off the electricity in your bedroom walls at night)

Question #6

How will you use and carry your cell phone and mobile electronic devices to minimize your direct exposure to the microwave radiation that they generate?

(See Chapter 6 for plenty of pointers.)

Question #7

When will you make time to unplug from the world of technology and re-connect with nature, yourself, and the people who are most important in your life?

(This could be as simple as taking a walk outdoors, spending some quiet, reflective time away from all of your technology, or engaging in a stimulating face-to-face conversation with a friend or family member.)

Question #8

If you could share just one idea in this book with another person, what would it be and who would you share it with?

(Sharing what you learn will not only enrich the lives of others but will enable you to more deeply embrace the learning yourself.)

Helpful Resources

Suppliers of EMF Safety Products and Devices

Less EMF Inc.
The EMF Safety Superstore
www.lessemf.com
1-888-537-7363
Meters, detectors, and protective shielding

The EMF Safety Store
www.emfsafetystore.com
EMF safety information, devices, and meters

Neuert Electromagnetic Services
http://www.emfcenter.com/metrsale.htm
1-800-638-3781
EMF shielding, devices, and meters for rental or sale

Stetzer Electric, Inc.
http://www.stetzerelectric.com/
Stetzerizer electric filters and micro-surge meter

EMF Solutions (Canada)
www.emfsolutions.ca/

Harmonizing devices for the home and office:

Advanced Living Technology
http://advancedlivingcomfort.com/
866-317-5683

Dimensional Design Products, Inc.
http://www.safespaceprotection.com/
866-821-8122

Educational Web Sites

The BioInitiative Report 2012:
The Rational for Biologically-Based Public Exposure
Standards for Electromagnetic Fields
www.bioinitiative.org
A 1479 page report by 29 distinguished and highly
recognized EMF experts.

Electric Sense
www.electricsense.com
Provides valuable advice on managing electromagnetic
stress. Features book reviews, articles by EMF experts, and
recorded expert interviews.

Electromagnetic Health
www.electromagnetichealth.com
Showcases audio clips and videos from leading EMF
experts.

World Health Organization
www.who.int/peh-emf/en/
Findings of the World Health Organization's International
EMF Project, which assesses the scientific evidence of the
possible health effects of EMFs.

Zapped
www.areyouzapped.com
Articles and updates about electro-pollution, EMF meters,
protective devices, and supplements to protect and heal
your body from electromagnetic stress.

EMF Consultants and Remediation Experts

International Institute for Building-Biology and Ecology
Listing of building biologists certified by the IBE:
http://hbelc.org/findexpert/enviroconsult
1-866-960-0333

Lloyd's List (compiled by Lloyd Burrell of Electric Sense)
http://www.electricsense.com/3125/emf-consultants-list/

Safe Living Technologies
Listing of EMF experts (USA, Canada & International)
www.slt.co/Company/EMFMitigationServiceProviders.aspx

My Top-Recommended EMF Expert for New Jersey and
the Surrounding Area (PA, New York City, etc.):

Sal La Duca
Environmental Assay, Inc.
Phillipsburg, NJ 08865
www.emfrelief.com
(908) 454-3965

In this book, I included an overview of the electrical
assessment of my home conducted by Sal La Duca. His
extensive knowledge of electrical environmental matters,
though, went far beyond anything I could describe. Thus, I
am confident in giving him my highest recommendation.

Total Body Modification
A natural healthcare technique used to neutralize the
negative effects of electromagnetic stress. For a list of
practitioners, go to www.tbmseminars.com.

Bibliography

Becker, Robert O., M.D. and Selden, Gary, *The Body Electric: Electromagnetism and Foundation of Life*, NY: William Morrow and Company Inc., 1985.

Blank, Martin, PhD, *Overpowered: What Science Tells Us About the Dangers of Cell Phones and Other Wifi-Age Devices*, NY: Seven Stories Press, 2014.

Crofton, Kerry, PhD, *Wireless Radiation Rescue: Safeguarding Your Family from the Risks of Electro-pollution*, Global WellBeing Books, 2010.

Davis, Devra, *Disconnect: The Truth About Cell Phone Radiation, What the Industry is Doing to Hide It, and How to Protect Your Family*, NY: Penguin Group, 2010.

Gittleman, Ann Louise, *Zapped: Why Your Cell Phone Shouldn't be Your Alarm Clock and 1268 Ways to Outsmart the Hazards of Electronic Pollution*, NY: HarperCollins Publishers, 2010.

Magee, Steven, *Toxic Electricity*, Edition 2, 2013.

Milham, Samuel, MD, MPH, *Dirty Electricity: Electrification and the Diseases of Civilization*, Bloomington, IN: iUniverse, 2010.

Singer, Katie, *An Electronic Silent Spring: Facing the Dangers and Creating Safe Limits*, Great Barrington, MA: Portal Books, 2014

About the Author

Sam Wieder specializes in working with chiropractors, fitness coaches, and other natural health professionals who are passionate advocates for healthy living. He helps his clients learn to speak with confidence and harness the power of their personal stories to motivate people to take command of their health.

Active in the world of public speaking for over 30 years, Sam has delivered numerous motivational presentations for professional audiences, conducted stress management workshops for office workers, and taught an environmental stress management seminar at an international health conference in Europe. His not-so-secret weapon for bringing all of these programs to life has been his personal stories, which he uses as both teaching metaphors and vehicles for moving his listeners to action.

As both a trainer and coach, Sam has coached a high school speech and debate team, taught college business communication classes, and led "Speak and Win Clients" groups for independent professionals. A Certified Trainer of Neuro-linguistic Programming, he brings to his work an understanding of the power of language and metaphor to create positive change in people's thinking and behavior.

Sam's greatest challenge in life has been his long-time struggle with the invisible assailant of electromagnetic stress. Yet by finally bringing that challenge to light and learning how to overcome it, he has uncovered a story that he believes is the most powerful and timely one that he has ever wanted to share. That story is the heart of this book.

Help the World to Unplug

Join me in my mission to educate people about the simple steps they can take to reduce fatigue and stay healthy in our high-tech world.

Healthcare Professionals

Offer your patients a copy of Unplug to empower them to take more responsibility for their health between office visits. Unplug makes a great patient appreciation gift.

Health and Safety-Conscious Employers

If your employees are heavy users of computers, cell phones, and other electronics, give them each a copy of Unplug to offer them a quick read that can make a big difference in their long-term health and productivity.

Passionate Advocates of Healthy Living

Send or give Unplug to your relatives, friends, and business contacts to show that you care. This is one book that they can read in about an hour to open the door to a lifetime of better health.

For details on quantity discounts, contact Sam Wieder at (724) 832-7459 or sam@CommandingConfidence.com.

CPSIA information can be obtained
at www.ICGtesting.com
Printed in the USA
LVOW10s1444120517

534313LV00010B/703/P